HEALING OSTEOARTHRITIS MADE SIMPLE

A COMPLETE GUIDE TO TREATMENT OF OSTEOARTHRITIS

DR. ALEXA LOWE

Table of Contents

CHAPTER ONE

treatment for osteoarthritis

Arthritis is a term used to describe changes in joint biomechanics. One of the most common forms of arthritis is osteoarthritis (OA). Osteoarthritis is caused by a variety of factors, including age.

What causes osteoarthritis?

By far, osteoarthritis (also referred to as DJD) is the most prevalent form of arthritis. A person's risk of developing osteoarthritis rises with age. Typically, the changes in osteoarthritis occur slowly over a long period of time, but there are exceptions. Joint inflammation and injury can lead to bone changes, deterioration of tendons and ligaments, as well as the breakdown of cartilage, resulting in pain, swelling, and deformity.

Fingers and thumbs are the most commonly affected parts of the body; the spine is also a common target as are hips, knees, and the great (little) toes.

Preexisting joint abnormalities, such as injury or trauma, such as repetitive or sports-related; rheumatoid, psoriatic or gout; infectious arthritis; genetic, congenital, or metabolic joint disorders; and metabolic joint abnormalities are all examples of secondary joint abnormalities that can occur.

What is cartilage, and how does it help the body?

Connective tissue known as cartilage covers the ends of bones in healthy joints. It is primarily composed of water and proteins and serves primarily as a "shock absorber" in the joints. Normal cartilage has a high water content, which allows it to change shape when compressed, making it a good shock absorber. Despite the fact that damaged cartilage can be repaired, the body does not produce new cartilage following an injury. Avascular: Cartilage does not have any blood vessels within it. As a result, recovery proceeds at a glacial pace.

Chondrocytes, the cartilage cells, and the matrix, a gel-like substance primarily composed of water and two types of proteins, make up cartilage (collagen and proteoglycans).

These cells, chondrocytes and their precursor chondroblasts, are extremely complex and multifunctional cartilage cells.

Cohesive extracellular matrix (ECM) components such as collagen and proteoglycans are essential for the growth and healing of healthy joints.

In addition to skin, tendons, and bone, collagen is found in cartilage and is an important structural protein. Cartilage's strength and structure are both attributed to collagen.

In cartilage, the complex molecules known as proteoglycans are made up of proteins and sugars that are intertwined. They act as a shock absorber by allowing cartilage to change shape when compressed by trapping large amounts of water. Proteoglycans, on the other hand, act as a repellent to each other, allowing cartilage to maintain its shape and elasticity.

Osteoarthritis affects whom?

Osteoarthritis is found in about 80% of people over the age of 55, according to an X-ray. Nearly two-thirds of those surveyed report some sort of ailment. Osteoarthritis affects an estimated 240 million adults worldwide, including more than

30 million adults in the United States. Compared to men, post-menopausal women are more likely to develop knee osteoarthritis than their male counterparts.

Osteoarthritis is caused by what?

Another factor that increases a person's risk of osteoarthritis is their genetic make-up. This can be inherited or influenced by other factors such as inflammatory arthritis or previous trauma.

Osteoarthritis, particularly in the knee, is exacerbated by obesity. Studies have found that obesity's metabolic and pro-inflammatory effects, in addition to overloading the body's weight-bearing mechanisms, play a role in osteoarthritis. Maintaining a healthy weight, or losing weight if necessary, is critical for those who are vulnerable.

Inflammation in the body can be exacerbated by diabetes and elevated lipids/cholesterol, both of which contribute to the development of osteoarthritis.

CHAPTER TWO

In the same way that atherosclerosis affects blood vessels, oxidation of lipids can produce deposits in cartilage that impair blood flow to subchondral bone. This oxidative stress exceeds the resilience of cartilage on the cellular level due to elevated blood sugars and elevated cholesterol/lipids. Along with overall health, maintaining healthy blood sugar and lipid levels is critical for strong bones.

Osteoarthritis of the knee is more likely in postmenopausal

women because estrogen protects bone health by reducing oxidative stress on cartilage. •

Osteoarthritis can run in families, as people with other bone diseases or genetic traits may be more prone to the condition. Osteoarthritis can be exacerbated by conditions such as Ehlers-Danlos, which is characterized by joint laxity or hypermobility.

Causes and Symptoms

Osteoarthritis is a multifactorial disease, not just "wear and tear" arthritis, because it has a variety of causes. Some of the factors that contribute to OA can be changed, while others cannot (cannot be changed such as born with it or now permanent). Osteoarthritis is more common in older people, but not everyone who has it experiences joint pain. Osteoarthritis can be exacerbated by inflammatory and metabolic factors, particularly in the presence of diabetes and/or elevated cholesterol.

In both primary and secondary forms, such as nodular OA of the hands or hypermobility of joints, osteoarthritis can be passed down through the family. Osteoarthritis secondary to chronic inflammation and joint destruction can result from infectious or inflammatory arthritis. Osteoarthritis can be aggravated by previous injuries or trauma, including sports-related or repetitive motion-related ones.

There have been recent advances in understanding the mechanisms of cartilage loss and bone changes, despite the fact that the exact mechanisms are still not known. Inflammation of the joints and faulty repair mechanisms in response to injury are thought to be the primary causes of cartilage degradation over time. Joint pain occurs as a result of activity because of other changes in the joint that cause it to lose mobility and function.

Osteoarthritis: How can I tell if I have it?

It takes months or years for the pain associated with osteoarthritis to develop, unlike other forms of arthritis. Running or prolonged walking, for example, can lead to an increase in pain in the joint. Swelling and pain in the joints tend to build up over time. A grinding or crunching sensation may be felt in the joints of those with advanced disease. In contrast to inflammatory arthritides, such as rheumatoid or psoriatic arthritis, morning stiffness is not a common symptom in OA. Osteoarthritis typically does not cause fevers, weight loss, or very red and hot joints. These signs and symptoms point to a different form of arthritis.

Osteoarthritis can usually be diagnosed by your healthcare provider (MD, DO, NP, PA) by getting a complete history of your symptoms and checking your joints. X-rays can help rule out any other potential causes of the discomfort. If a cartilage or surrounding ligament tear is suspected, an MRI may be warranted. Otherwise, it is not routinely required. Osteoarthritis cannot be diagnosed using blood tests. A doctor may have to drain fluid from a swollen joint if that joint is particularly swollen. The fluid can be tested for signs of other types of arthritis, such as gout, by conducting tests.

PROPERTY MANAGEMENT AND HEALTH CARE

The treatment for osteoarthritis is what?

Osteoarthritis is incurable. When symptoms are mild to moderate, a combinationof pharmacological and non-pharmacological approaches usually works well. In terms of medical care and advice, some options are as follows:

Prescription Drugs (topical pain medicines and oral analgesics including nonsteroidal anti-inflammatory medications, NSAIDs).

• Workout (land- and water-based).

Use of alternately hot and cold compresses (local modalities).

- Physiotherapy, occupational therapy, and exercise therapy are all included in this category.

Reduced body mass (if overweight).

- Diabetes and cholesterol management.

Braces, orthotics, shoe inserts or a cane are examples of supportive devices.

intra-articular steroid and hyaluronic acid "gel" injections

Vitamins and supplements are one type of complementary and alternative medicine.

When other medical options have failed or have been exhausted, surgery may be an option to alleviate pain and restore function.

The following are the intended outcomes of treatment:

• Delay the progression of joint pain and stiffness.

Achieve greater ease of movement and improved performance.

• Improve the quality of life for patients.

The patient's age, general health, daily activities, occupation, and the severity of the condition all play a role in determining the type of treatment regimen prescribed.

CHAPTER THREE

Osteoarthritis has made much slower progress than other types of arthritis, which have seen significant advances in the last few years. Osteoarthritis cannot be reversed or slowed down by any medications currently on the market.. As of now, medication is focused on alleviating symptoms. Acetaminophen and nonsteroidal anti-inflammatory drugs (NSAIDs) are common pain relievers (NSAIDs). Tolerance and addiction to narcotic painkillers are possible because of the chronic nature of the disease. Applying analgesic patches, creams, rubs or sprays directly to the skin of the affected area can help alleviate discomfort.

Osteoarthritis sufferers should consult a doctor before taking any of these medications, even if they are available over the counter. Medication interactions and/or side effects, whether dangerous or unwanted, are common occurrences. There are still some over-the-counter medications that need to be tested in the lab on an ongoing basis.

Pain from osteoarthritis, such as lower back pain, can be treated with the antidepressant duloxetine hydrochloride which was approved by the FDA in 2010. For those who are unable to take NSAIDs or other medications, this has been a lifesaver.

Assistive technologies

Reduced joint stress can be alleviated using supportive or assistive devices. Joints that have been damaged or injured can be supported and stabilized by braces and orthotics. When using a medical device, always follow the directions provided by a healthcare professional such as a physical or occupational therapist or your licensed physician's office. Using a cane or a walker, a shoe lift/insert, or some other walking aid can help relieve pressure on certain joints and improve body and gait mechanics.

Exercise

Flexibility, joint stability, and muscle strength can all be improved with regular exercise. Recommendations include low-impact exercises such as swimming and water aerobics. They've been shown to reduce pain and disability in osteoarthritis sufferers. Excessively strenuous exercise programs should be avoided, as they may worsen arthritis symptoms and potentially speed up the disease's progression. For those suffering from osteoarthritis, physical or occupational therapists can help devise an exercise plan that is both safe and effective.

The use of alternately hot and cold methods of treatment

Temporary relief from pain and stiffness may be achieved by using hot and cold treatments. A hot shower or bath, as well as the careful application of heating or cooling pads or packs, are examples of these treatments.

control of one's weight

Work on weight management may help prevent and improve

osteoarthritis, which is known to be associated with obesity. Stress and pain in weight-bearing joints can be reduced and inflammation can be moderated by weight loss in overweight people with osteoarthritis.

Surgery

Surgical intervention may be necessary when the pain of osteoarthritis is so severe that it interferes with daily activities. Surgeons typically perform surgery only on patients with severe osteoarthritis. Joint replacement surgery can be performed using a variety of methods, including minimally invasive ones. For the right patients, joint surgery can be extremely beneficial in terms of restoring some function and alleviating pain.

Medicine that isn't conventional

Alternate medicine, as well as supplements As a term derived from "nutrition and pharmaceutical," nutraceuticals are compounds that can be purchased without a prescription from pharmacies or health food stores and are not approved by the FDA as drugs. The term "natural," "homeopathic," or "alternative" therapies can encompass a wide range of substances, including dietary supplements, vitamins, minerals, and other compounds. A wide variety of formulations are available, the amount of active ingredients may vary, and the label and product accuracy cannot be guaranteed because this market is less regulated than the food or pharmaceutical industry.

Normal cartilage contains the amino acids glucosamine and chondroitin. Sulfate compounds are the most common form in which they are sold as a dietary supplement. Some studies suggest that glucosamine and chondroitin may have pain-relieving properties, particularly in osteoarthritis of the knee. However, clinical research results seem to vary. Even if they do work, it's still unclear how they do it, and there's no solid scientific evidence to back up the claim that they do. To be safe, you should first consult with your doctor before taking glucosamine and chondroitin supplements.

For rheumatoid arthritis, fish oils have been found to have some anti-inflammatory properties. Because of the possibility of drug interactions and possible side effects, it is always advisable to discuss dietary supplements with your doctor before taking them.

Acupuncture, acupressure, and meditation are all forms of complementary and alternative medicine.

THE END